KEY TA

ANAESTHESIA AND
INTENSIVE CARE

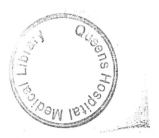

KEY FACTS IN ANAESTHESIA AND INTENSIVE CARE

Alcira Serrano Gomez
MD Fellow
John Farman Intensive Care Unit
Addenbrooke's NHS Trust
Cambridge, UK

Gilbert R Park
MD DMed Sci FRCA
Director of Intensive Care Research
John Farman Intensive Care Unit
Addenbrooke's NHS Trust
Cambridge, UK

LONDON • SAN FRANCISCO

Project Manager
Gavin Smith

Typeset by Charon Tec Pvt. Ltd, Chennai, India

Printed in the UK by The Alden Group Ltd, Oxford

Distributed by Plymbridge Distributors Ltd and
in the USA by Jamco Distribution

Visit our website at www.greenwich-medical.co.uk

CONTENTS

PREFACE TO
SECOND EDITION

The aim of this booklet is to be a readily available source of information and guidance for junior medical staff working in intensive care or anaesthesia. It is impossible to include all the information each clinician may require, so it is our intention that individuals add to, or subtract information from, this booklet as necessary.

Dosages have been included for many drugs; despite careful checking, mistakes may have occurred and, if a dose appears incorrect, it should be checked with the package insert, *British National Formulary* or other suitable reference source, before the drug is administered.

We gratefully acknowledge the assistance and co-operation of the many medical, nursing, laboratory, measurement and other paramedical personnel, from whom we have received numerous helpful suggestions during the preparation of this booklet.

We would be grateful for the readers' comments or suggestions for future editions.

GR Park
RJ Kavanagh
Cambridge, 1995

PREFACE TO THIRD EDITION

Seven years have passed since the last edition of this little pocket book. Clearly, it is time for an update. This edition incorporates not only our ideas of what is needed, but also the many helpful comments we have received from the readers of our previous edition.

The aim of the book remains unchanged, to provide doctors, nurses, physiotherapists and others with clear concise information. Many readers do have ideas on how we can improve the book further, we would be pleased to hear from them.

The guidelines within this book are not to be construed as standards of medical care. These are determined on the basis of all clinical data available for an individual patient and will change as knowledge advances.

The ultimate decision about a treatment plan or procedure for a patient must be made in the light of all the clinical information and the possible diagnostic and treatments available. However, we hope this book will provide some help with this.

Alcira Serrano Gomez
Gilbert Park
Cambridge, 2002

To our friends and colleagues around the world – thank you.

COMMON ABBREVIATIONS

ABG	arterial blood gases
AF	atrial fibrillation
CI	cardiac index
cal	calories
CJD	Creutzfeldt–Jakob disease
CK	creatine kinase
CNS	central nervous system
CO	cardiac output
CPK	creatine phosphokinase
CrCl	creatinine clearance
CVP	central venous pressure
CXR	chest X-ray
CT	computed tomogram
DIC	disseminated intravascular coagulation
dL	decilitre
ECG	electrocardiogram
EDTA	ethylenediaminetetraacetic acid
EMD	electromechanical dissociation
EMLA	eutectic mixture of local anaesthetic
FBC	full blood count
FDPs	fibrin-degradation products
FFP	fresh frozen plasma
F_iO_2	fractional inspired oxygen concentration
h	hour
Hb	haemoglobin
HAS	human albumin solution
HIV	human immunodeficiency virus
IM	intramuscularly
IPPV	intermittent positive pressure ventilation
iu	international unit
IV	intravenously
J	Joule

K^{++}	potassium
kg	kilogram
kcal	kilocalories
kPa	kilopascals
KPTT	kaolin partial thromboplastin time
L	litre
LDH	lactate dehydrogenase
μg	micrograms
MAC	minimum alveolar concentration
MAP	mean arterial pressure
MCH	mean cell haemoglobin
MCV	mean cell volume
Mg^{++}	magnesium
mL	millilitre
mmol	millimole
μmol	micromole
MPAP	mean pulmonary arterial pressure
MRSA	methicillin-resistant *Staphylococcus aureus*
N_2O	nitrous oxide
NG	nasogastric
O	orally
O_2	oxygen
P_aCO_2	partial pressure of carbon dioxide in blood
PAFC	pulmonary arterial flotation catheter
P_aO_2	partial presssure of oxygen in blood
PEA	pulseless electrical activity
PCV	packed cell volume
PCWP	pulmonary capillary wedge pressure
PR	per rectum
PT	prothrombin time
S_aO_2	arterial oxygen saturation
S_vO_2	mixed venous oxygen saturation
SVR	systemic vascular resistance
TPN	total parenteral nutrition
TT	thrombin time
VE	ventricular extrasystoles
VF	ventricular fibrillation
WCC	white cell count
Zn	zinc

For haemodynamic variables, see page 21

USEFUL TELEPHONE NUMBERS

Laboratories
    Biochemistry ....
    Haematology ....
    Transfusion ....
    Microbiology ....

Theatres
    Reception ....
    Recovery ....
    ....
    ....
    ....

Imaging
    Portable XR ....
    CT ....
    Ultrasound ....

Wards
    Intensive Care ....
    Coronary Care ....
    ....
    ....
    ....
    ....
    ....
    ....

Services
    Porters ....
    Transplant Coordinator ....
    Poisons Unit ....

Others
  Medic Alert Foundation   0800581420
  Malignant hyperthermia
    Direct line   0113 206 5274
    Fax   0113 206 4140
    Emergency 'hotline' bleep   0345 333 111 No. 0525 420
  Guys poison unit   0870 600 6266
  UK Transplant and Organ
    Donor Register   0845 60 60 400

NORMAL VALUES

BIOCHEMISTRY

	Normal range
Blood: Urea and electrolytes	
Sodium	132–142 mmol/L
Potassium	3.4–5 mmol/L
Bicarbonate	22–30 mmol/L
Glucose	3.5–7 mmol/L
Urea	<7.5 mmol/L
Creatinine	35–125 μmol/L
Chloride	95–106 mmol/L
Osmolality	280–300 mosmol/kg
Liver function tests	
Total protein	63–83 g/L
Albumin	30–44 g/L
Bilirubin	2–17 μmol/L
Alkaline phosphatase	30–135 U/L
Alanine aminotransferase	7–40 U/L
Total calcium	2.2–2.6 mmol/L
Ionised calcium	1.18–1.30 mmol/L
Phosphate	0.8–1.4 mmol/L
Zinc	12–23 μmol/L
Magnesium	0.7–1.0 mmol/L
Arterial blood gases	
Hydrogen ion	36–45 nmol/L
pH	7.36–7.44
P_aCO_2	4.7–6 kPa
P_aO_2	9.3–14 kPa
Base excess	±2.5 mmol/L
Standard bicarbonate	21–25 mmol/L
Urine	
Sodium	50–200 mmol/24 h
Potassium	20–60 mmol/24 h

Continued

BIOCHEMISTRY (*continued*)

	Normal range
Urea	330–500 mmol/24 h
Creatinine	9–16 mmol/24 h
Protein	<0.1 g/24 h
Creatinine clearance	90–120 mL/min
Osmolality	300–1200 mosmol/kg

HAEMATOLOGY

	Normal range
Haemoglobin	
Men	14.0–17.0 g/dL
Women	11.5–16.0 g/dL
Platelet count	$150–300 \times 10^9$/L
White cell count (WCC)	$4.0–11 \times 10^9$/L
Differential white counts	
Neutrophils	$2.0–7.5 \times 10^9$/L (40–75% of WCC)
Lymphocytes	$1.5–4.4 \times 10^9$/L (20–40% of WCC)
Monocytes	$0.2–0.8 \times 10^9$/L (2–10% of WCC)
Eosinophils	$0.04–0.4 \times 10^9$/L (1–6% of WCC)
Basophils	$<0.1 \times 10^9$/L (<1% of WCC)
Prothrombin time (PT)	<2 s above control
Kaolin partial thromboplastin time (KPTT)	<7 s above control
Fibrinogen	1.5–4.0 g/L
Fibrin-degradation products (FDPs)	<0.5 mg/L

USEFUL CALCULATED VALUES

Osmolality

Plasma:

   osmolality (mosmol/kg) = $[2 \times (Na + K)]$ + urea + glucose

Urine:

   osmolality (mosmol/kg) = $[2 \times (Na + K)]$ + urea − 10

Creatinine clearance

$$\text{Creatinine clearance (mL/min)} = \frac{\text{Urine creatinine (mmol/24 h)} \times 694}{\text{Plasma creatinine (}\mu\text{mol/L)}}$$

Nitrogen balance

Nitrogen output (g/24 h) = (urine urea $\times$ 0.035)
$$+ (\Delta \text{ plasma urea} \times \text{body weight (kg)} \times 0.046)$$

where Δ plasma urea is the difference between one day's result and the previous day's.

RESUSCITATION

ADULT CARDIAC ARREST FLOW CHART

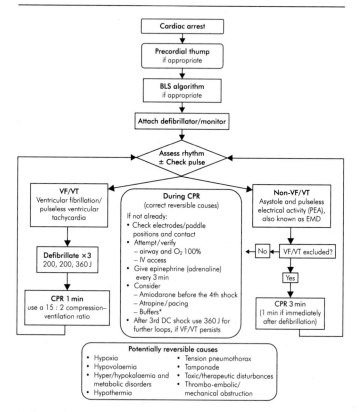

* Buffers: Sodium bicarbonate, if pH <7.1 (H⁺ >80 mmol/L) and/or cardiac arrest
associated with tricyclic overdose or hyperkalaemia

Footnote continued

The number of times the loop is repeated is a matter of clinical judgement. If it was appropriate to start resuscitation, it is usually considered worthwhile continuing as long as the patient remains in identifiable VF/VT

Chest compression and simultaneous ventilation at 12 breaths/min may offer advantages in the intubated patient

Bingham R, Handley A, Evans T, Nolan J, Phillips B, Richmond S and Wyllie J. *Resuscitation Guidelines*. Resuscitation Council, London. 2000

CARDIAC ARREST DRUGS AND DOSES

All doses based on a 70 kg patient.

Drug	Intravenous (IV) dose
Epinephrine (Adrenaline)	1 mg (10 mL of 1 : 10,000)
Atropine[a]	3 mg
Amiodarone	150 mg (made up to 20 mL with 5% glucose)
	150 mg further doses for recurrent or refractory VF/VT
	Infusion of 1 mg/min for 6 h and then 0.5 mg/min to a maximum of 2 g in 24 h
Lidocaine[b] (Lignocaine)	100 mg (1–1.5 mg/kg)
	50 mg additional bolus; not exceed 3 mg/kg in the 1st hour
Magnesium[c]	8 mmol
Sodium bicarbonate	50 mL of 8.4%
Calcium chloride[d]	10 mL of 10% (6.8 mmol)

[a] Atropine should be given in asystole and PEA associated with a bradycardia (<60/min)
[b] Lidocaine should not be given if the patient has received amiodarone; but may be used as an alternative, if amiodarone is not available
[c] Magnesium should be given for refractory VF, if there is any suspicion of hypomagnesaemia
[d] Calcium indicated in PEA caused by hyperkalaemia, hypocalcaemia or overdose of calcium-channel-blocking drugs; may be repeated if necessary

Intra-tracheal drug doses and administration

Dilute the drug in 10–20 mL of 0.9% saline and inject into the tracheo-bronchial tree using a suction catheter inserted through the tracheal tube. *Only use for* epinephrine, lidocaine and atropine, at 2–2.5 times the IV dose.

Drug	Intra-tracheal dose (mg)
Epinephrine (Adrenaline)	2–3
Atropine	6
Lidocaine (Lignocaine)	200

Bingham R, Handley A, Evans T, Nolan J, Phillips B, Richmond S and Wyllie J. *Resuscitation Guidelines*. Resuscitation Council, London. 2000

PAEDIATRIC CARDIAC ARREST FLOW CHART

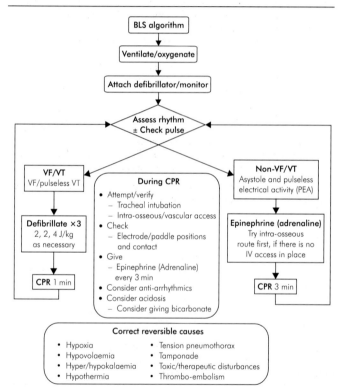

Bingham R, Handley A, Evans T, Nolan J, Phillips B, Richmond S and Wyllie J. *Resuscitation Guidelines*. Resuscitation Council, London. 2000

PAEDIATRIC CARDIAC ARREST DRUGS AND DOSES

Most cardiac arrests in children are secondary to hypoxia caused by respiratory failure. Hypovolaemia is the second most common cause, caused either to blood loss or loss of body fluids (e.g. dehydration secondary to gastroenteritis). Primary cardiac arrest caused by heart disease is rare.

- *External cardiac massage:* For an infant (child <1-year old) locate the sternum and place the tips of two fingers, one finger's breadth below an imaginary line joining the infant's nipples. Press down on the sternum to depress it approximately one-third to one-half of the infant's chest at a rate of 100 compressions per minute. In older children, place the heel of one hand over the lower half of the sternum. The compression to ventilation ratio should be 5 : 1.
- *Epinephrine large doses:* There is no convincing evidence that a second and subsequent dose of epinephrine of 100 μg/kg IV is beneficial. However, there are some cases of return of spontaneous circulation with large doses of epinephrine; therefore, if the patient has a continuous intra-arterial monitoring, the dose can be titrated to best effect.
- *IV fluids:* When the cardiac arrest has resulted from circulatory failure, a standard (20 mL/kg) bolus of crystalloid fluid should be given, if there is no response to the initial dose of epinephrine.
- *Amiodarone:* The dose of amiodarone for VF/pulseless VT is followed by continued CPR and a further defibrillation attempt within 60 s.

After each drug, CPR should continue for up to 1 min to allow the drug to reach the heart before a further defibrillation attempt.

Drug doses for children

Drug	IV dose
Adenosine	0.1 mg/kg
Epinephrine (Adrenaline)	10 μg/kg (0.1 mL/kg of 1 : 10,000)
Atropine	0.02 mg/kg
Amiodarone	5 mg/kg
Sodium bicarbonate*	1 mL/kg of an 8.4% solution
Calcium chloride (10%)	0.2–0.25 mL/kg
Naloxone	10 μg/kg

* In patients with prolonged cardiac arrest or cardiac arrest associated with documented severe metabolic acidosis

Intra-tracheal drug doses and administration

Ten times the IV dose should be given through this route. The drug should be injected quickly down a narrow bore suction catheter beyond the tracheal end of the tube and then flushed in with 1 or 2 mL of 0.9% saline. The second and subsequent doses should be given at 2–2.5 times the IV dose.

Drug	Intra-tracheal dose
Epinephrine (adrenaline)	100 μg/kg (1 mL/kg of 1 : 10,000)
Atropine	0.2 mg/kg

Bingham R, Handley A, Evans T, Nolan J, Phillips B, Richmond S and Wyllie J. *Resuscitation Guidelines.* Resuscitation Council, London. 2000

RESUSCITATION FROM SHOCK

Shock is a common emergency encountered in the critically ill and during anaesthesia. It may be caused by one of the following:

- hypovolaemia,
- sepsis,
- pump failure (cardiogenic shock),
- anaphylaxis.

Remember that several causes for shock may exist at the same time in the same patient. There are certain common steps in all types of shock. Several steps may need to be done concurrently:

- Ensure adequate ventilation and oxygenation. It is safer artificially to ventilate the patient early, if respiratory insufficiency is clinically evident, than wait until severe respiratory failure becomes apparent.
- Establish venous access.
- Monitoring
  - continuous ECG display;
  - arterial catheter;
  - central venous pressure (CVP) measurement;
  - urinary catheter and hourly output measurement.
- Give adequate analgesia, if the patient is in pain. Small doses of morphine (1–2 mg) should be given IV every 3 min until the pain is relieved.

Hypovolaemic shock

Caused by excessive loss of fluid from the body: blood, plasma or salt and water, it should be treated with intravascular volume expansion with an appropriate fluid.

If the patient has lost blood, it should be replaced with whole blood or a mixture of concentrated red cells and a crystalloid (e.g. Hartmann's or Ringers lactate) or a colloid solution (e.g. gelatin or starch). When a mixture of blood and exudate is lost (e.g. after abdominal surgery), the haematocrit should be measured after every 2 L of fluid and maintained at about 0.3 using a mixture of blood, gelatin or starch solution, etc. Hypovolaemia from other causes should be treated initially with plasma volume expansion.

Adequacy of volume replacement can be gauged by a decreasing heart rate, increasing blood pressure and urine output, and warming of the peripheries. The CVP or PAFC offers further guidance.

Once intravascular volume has been restored other fluids can be given, as necessary, to replace extravascular fluid losses, such as those seen in dehydration.

Cardiogenic shock

This follows myocardial damage by ischaemia, infarction or myocardial toxins. The patient is peripherally shut down and cyanosed. As the myocardium is damaged, the CVP may not give an accurate reflection of left-sided filling pressures, and the insertion of a pulmonary arterial flotation catheter is invaluable in assessing whether hyper- or hypovolaemia is present. Cardiac output may also be measured allowing the rational choice of drug therapy.

Treatment

1. Correct any arrhythmias (see page 13).
2. Inotropic support (see page 12).
3. Afterload reduction. Decreases the amount of work done by a damaged heart. This can be achieved by using a vasodilator such as sodium nitroprusside or a combined inotrope/dilator such as dopexamine.

Septic shock

Septic shock can be caused by any organism, but is most commonly caused by Gram-negative bacteria. Three components may contribute to cardiovascular dysfunction in septic shock:

1. In the early stages, peripheral vasodilation may occur, with a low systemic vascular resistance (SVR). Later, vasoconstriction occurs with a markedly increased SVR.
2. Hypovolaemia: the capillaries leak and allow protein-rich fluid to leak into the tissues, particularly the lungs.

3. Myocardial depression caused by the combined effects of bacterial toxins and a metabolic acidosis.

Treatment

1. Antibiotics after blood cultures and other relevant specimens have been taken.
2. Restoration of circulating blood volume with a colloid solution with guidance from CVP measurements, in cold septic shock, or in those who develop pulmonary or renal dysfunction.
3. Inotropic support of a depressed myocardium initially using epinephrine (see page 12).
4. Manipulation of the SVR (measured using a pulmonary artery flotation catheter).

Anaphylactic shock

Clinical features of anaphylaxis (% frequency)

- Cardiovascular collapse (88%)
- Bronchospasm (36%)
- Angio-oedema commonly of the face, e.g. periorbital and perioral (24%)
- Generalised oedema (7%)
- Cutaneous signs such as rash (13%), erythema (45%) and urticaria (8.5%)

First clinical features in severe reactions (% frequency)

- No pulse detected, decrease in arterial pressure (28%)
- Difficult to inflate lungs (26%)
- Flush (21%)
- Coughing (6%)
- Rash (4%)
- Desaturation (3%)
- Cyanosis (3%)
- Others (e.g. ECG changes, urticaria, swelling) (9%)

Investigation

No tests that can be performed at the time of the reaction have been shown to provide useful information for immediate clinical management.

Approximately 1 h after the beginning of the reaction, 10 mL of venous blood should be taken into a glass tube. The serum should be separated and stored at −20°C until the sample can be sent to a reference laboratory for estimation of serum tryptase concentration. Elevated serum tryptase concentration indicates that the reaction was associated with mast cell degranulation. This may occur in both anaphylactic and anaphylactoid reactions. However, a negative test does not completely exclude anaphylaxis.

Treatment

Initial therapy

1. Stop administration of drug(s) likely to have caused the anaphylaxis.
2. Maintain airway: give 100% oxygen.
3. Lay patient flat with feet elevated.
4. Give epinephrine (adrenaline):
   - This may be given in a dose of 0.5–1 mg IM (0.5–1 mL of 1 : 1000) and may be repeated every 10 min according to the arterial pressure and pulse until improvement occurs.
   - Alternatively, 50–100 μg IV over 1 min has been recommended (0.5–1 mL of 1 : 10,000) for hypotension with titration of further doses as required.
   - In a patient with cardiovascular collapse, 0.5–1 mg (5–10 mL of 1 : 10,000) may be required IV in divided doses by titration. This should be given at a rate of 0.1 mg/min stopping when a response has been obtained.
5. Start intravascular volume expansion with crystalloid or colloid 10 mL/kg rapidly.

Secondary therapy

1. Antihistamines (chlorpheniramine 10–20 mg by slow IV infusion).
2. Corticosteroids (hydrocortisone 100–300 mg IV or methylprednisolone 2 g IV).
3. Catecholamine infusions (epinephrine or norepinephrine). See page 12 for doses.
4. Consider bicarbonate (0.5–1 mmol/kg IV) for acidosis.
5. Airway evaluation (before extubation).
6. Bronchodilators may be required for persistent bronchospasm. Consider:
   - Salbutamol 250 μg IV loading dose/5–20 μg/min maintenance,
   - Terbutaline 250–500 μg/min IV loading dose/1.5 μg/min maintenance, or
   - Aminophylline 6 μg/kg IV over 20 min.

Suspected Anaphylactic Reactions Associated with Anaesthesia, revised edition. Association of Anaesthetists in Great Britain and Ireland. 1995. www.aagbi.org/guidelines.html

VASOACTIVE DRUG INFUSIONS

The concentrations of drugs described here are for administration by syringe pump through a centrally placed venous line used solely for this purpose. If these criteria are not met, then dilute the same quantity of drug in 500 mL of 5% glucose and multiply the starting dose by 10.

The starting dose will require adjustment (increase or decrease) based on individual patient response. All doses based on a 70 kg adult patient.

Drug	Infusion dose (μg/kg/min)	Dilution made up to 50 mL 5% glucose	Starting dose (mL/h)
Epinephrine (Adrenaline)	0.025–0.25	5 mg = 100 μg/mL	1
Dobutamine	2.5–10	250 mg = 5000 μg/mL	2.1
Dopamine		200 mg = 4000 μg/mL	
Low dose	1–5		1
Moderate	5–10		5
Dopexamine	0.5–6	200 mg = 4000 μg/mL	0.5*
Glyceryl trinitrate	0.2–3	50 mg = 1000 μg/mL	0.8
Lidocaine (Lignocaine)	100 mg bolus 4 mg/min for 30 min 2 mg/min for 2 h then 1 mg/min	400 mg = 8 mg/mL	30–50
Norepinephrine (Noradrenaline)	0.02–0.4	16 mg = 320 μg/mL	2–3
Phenylephrine	1–5	25 mg = 500 μg/mL	8
Salbutamol	5 μg/min initially 3–20 μg/min	10 mg = 200 μg/mL	1.5
Sodium nitroprusside	10–200 μg/min	50 mg = 1000 μg/mL	0.6

*Anti-inflammatory use 0.5–1 mL/h
BNF 43, March 2002. www.bnf.org

WHICH VASOACTIVE AGENTS TO USE WHEN INCREASING CARDIAC INDEX, BLOOD PRESSURE, DO$_2$, ETC.

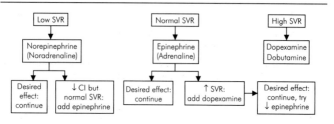

NORMAL CARDIOVASCULAR VARIABLES AND THEIR CALCULATION

Measured variables (mmHg)

Right atrium
  Mean   −1 to +7
Right ventricle
  Systolic   15–25
  End diastolic   0–8
Pulmonary artery
  Systolic   15–25
  Diastolic   8–15
  Mean (MPAP)   10–20
Pulmonary capillary wedge pressure
  Mean (PCWP)   6–12
Central venous pressure (CVP)   5–12

Derived variables (in mmHg)

$$\text{Mean arterial pressure (MAP)} = \text{diastolic} + \frac{(\text{systolic} - \text{diastolic})}{3}$$

See page 21 for more cardiovascular variables

TREATMENT OF ARRHYTHMIAS

If the patient's lungs are being ventilated check:

1. The ventilator is switched on.
2. The oxygen supply is functioning correctly (oxygen rotameters, air/oxygen blender).
3. There are no leaks or disconnections in the circuit.

Before treating arrhythmias ensure that

- the patient is not hypo- or hyperkalaemic,
- the patient is not hypoxic ($P_aO_2 < 8$ kPa),
- the patient is not hypercarbic ($P_aCO_2 > 6$ kPa),
- the patient is not distressed (in pain, etc.),
- the monitor is not wrongly connected,
- a CVP or PA catheter is not irritating the heart.

If the patient has a life-threatening tachyarrhythmia, consider immediate DC cardioversion before using drugs.

Always obtain a 12-lead ECG before and during pharmacological interventions and after conversion to a regular rhythm.

Never use more than one agent unless absolutely necessary. When an appropriate dose fails, use DC cardioversion rather than a second drug.

First line treatment of common arrhythmias

For drug doses, see page 15.

Ectopics

- Supraventricular
  - Treat only if causing haemodynamic instability.
  - Atenolol.
- Ventricular
  - There is no evidence that suppressing asymptomatic ventricular extrasystoles is worthwhile.
  - Correct precipitating causes.
  - Lidocaine bolus followed by infusion, if necessary (page 12).

Narrow-complex supraventricular tachycardia

- Attempt therapeutic diagnostic manoeuvre:
  - Carotid sinus massage. *Caution:* one side only at a time.
  - Adenosine.
- Amiodarone, β-blockers or calcium-channel blockers, if EF > 40%.
- If cardiac function is compromised (EF < 40%) use only amiodarone.
- Do not use DC cardioversion in patients with impaired cardiac function.

Atrial fibrillation/atrial flutter

- Haemodynamically unstable, rapid response needed: Heparanise and synchronised DC cardioversion (start with 100 J). Under sedation or general anaesthesia.
- Stable, impaired cardiac function (EF < 40%): digitalis, diltiazem or amiodarone.

Ventricular tachycardia

- DC cardioversion, if haemodynamically unstable or if drug therapy is ineffective.
- Correct acid–base and potassium abnormalities.
- If stable: amiodarone or lidocaine, then use synchronised cardioversion.

Ventricular fibrillation

- See 'Cardiac arrest flow chart' (page 4).

Heart block

- Stop drugs exacerbating or causing the conduction defect.
- The decision to pace is made on symptoms and haemodynamic effects, not the specific arrhythmia.
- Pacing is normally required on Mobitz type 2 and third-degree heart block following a myocardial infarct.

Some common anti-arrhythmic drug doses

Adenosine	6 mg bolus. If necessary, three further doses each of 12 mg every 1–2 min. Overuse of this drug is potentially dangerous
Amiodarone	150 mg (made up to 20 mL 5% glucose) over 10 min for stable tachyarrhythmias. 150 mg further doses Infusion of 1 mg/min for 6 h and then 0.5 mg/min to a maximum of 2 g in 24 h
Atenolol	2.5 mg (1 mg/min) IV repeated every 5 min. Maximum 10 mg
Digoxin	Loading dose 0.5 mg in 50 mL 5% glucose over 30 min, repeated once if necessary
Esmolol	40 mg (0.5 mg/kg) over 1 min, then infuse at 4 mg/min (0.05 mg/kg), if necessary increased gradually up to 0.1 mg/kg/min
Lidocaine (Lignocaine)	IV bolus of 50 mg (0.5–0.75 mg/kg), can be repeated every 5 min to a maximum of 200 mg
Verapamil	5–10 mg IV over 2 min. Further, 5 mg can be given 5 min later, if required

Special Issue Guidelines 2000 for cardiopulmonary resuscitation and emergency cardiovascular care – an international consensus on science. *Resuscitation* 2000; **46**(1–3): 135–53, 185–93

ECG paper

Vertical axis represents voltage. 10 mm = 1 mV
Horizontal axis represents speed. 1 mm = 0.04 s

ECG variables

PR interval	0.12–0.20 s
QRS complex	0.04–0.10 s
P wave	<0.11 s
QRS axis	$-30°$ to $+90°$

THE APPROACH TO THE BLEEDING PATIENT

The following questions should be asked:
- Is the patient adequately resuscitated?
- During massive transfusion have coagulation factors been replaced (see below)?
- Has the underlying cause been treated adequately, e.g. surgically correctable bleeding or sepsis?
- Have any drugs that alter coagulation been given within, or outside, the hospital (aspirin, heparin for monitoring lines)?
- Is there a past history or a family history of abnormal bleeding (haemophilia)? Has the patient a warning bracelet or card about drug therapy (oral anticoagulants) or disease?
- Does the patient suffer from a condition that interferes with vitamin K absorption (jaundice, malabsorption)?

Consult a haematologist with all coagulation problems.

Remove heparin from the monitoring flush lines until it is corrected.

THE ASSESSMENT OF BLEEDING DISORDERS

Investigations

- *Platelet count.* Significant if below 80×10^9/L.
- *Prothrombin time (PT).* Assesses the extrinsic and common pathway. Also used to guide warfarin dose.
- *Kaolin partial thromboplastin time (KPTT).* Assesses the intrinsic and common pathway. Used to guide heparin dosage.
- *Thrombin time (TT).* Assesses the conversion of fibrinogen to fibrin.
- *Plasma fibrinogen.* Assay of this factor.
- *Fibrin-degradation products (FDPs).* Increased when excessive fibrin is being broken down.

MASSIVE BLOOD TRANSFUSION

Platelet count reduced; PT and KPTT increased; TT, fibrinogen and FDPs normal. This occurs when more than one circulating blood volume has been replaced rapidly. In addition to the loss of platelets and clotting factors, citrate binds calcium and renders it inactive.

Treat on the basis of coagulation results. If not available give 2 U of fresh-frozen plasma (FFP) per 10 U of blood and also calcium gluconate (2.2 mmol IV) every 4 U of blood given. Platelet administration is based on the platelet count.

MANAGEMENT OF FAILED TRACHEAL INTUBATION

- Do not give another dose of muscle relaxant.
- Do not keep trying to intubate the trachea without oxygenating the patient using a mask and a self-inflating bag.
- Maintain cricoid pressure, if there is risk for regurgitation and aspiration.

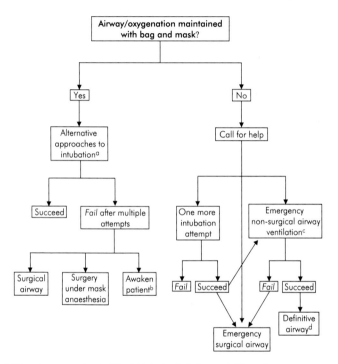

[a] Alternative approaches to difficult intubation include use of different laryngoscope blades, awake intubation, blind oral or nasal intubation, fibre-optic intubation, intubating stylet or tube changer, light wand and retrograde intubation

[b] See awake intubation page 18

[c] Options for emergency non-surgical airway ventilation include: trans-tracheal jet ventilation, laryngeal mask ventilation, or oesophageal–tracheal combitube ventilation

[d] Options for establishing a definitive airway include: returning to awake state with spontaneous ventilation, tracheotomy, or endotracheal intubation

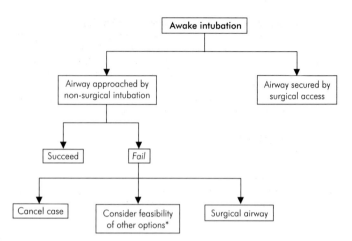

```
                    ┌─────────────────┐
                    │ Awake intubation │
                    └─────────────────┘
                             │
           ┌─────────────────┴─────────────────┐
  ┌──────────────────┐              ┌──────────────────┐
  │ Airway approached by │          │ Airway secured by │
  │ non-surgical intubation │       │ surgical access │
  └──────────────────┘              └──────────────────┘
           │
    ┌──────┴──────┐
┌─────────┐  ┌──────┐
│ Succeed │  │ Fail │
└─────────┘  └──────┘
                │
    ┌───────────┼──────────────┐
┌──────────┐ ┌──────────────┐ ┌────────────────┐
│Cancel case│ │Consider feasibility│ │Surgical airway│
└──────────┘ │ of other options* │ └────────────────┘
             └──────────────┘
```

* Other options include surgery under mask anaesthesia, surgery under local anaesthesia, or regional nerve blockade, or intubation attempts after induction of general anaesthesia.

Practice guidelines for Management of the Difficult Airway: A report by the American Society of Anesthesiologists Task Force on Management of the Difficult Airway. *Anesthesiology* 1993; **78**: 597 (www.asahq.org/publications and services).

ACCIDENTAL INTRA-ARTERIAL INJECTION

Signs

1. Immediate agonising pain spreading distally from site of injection.
2. Blanching caused by severe arterial spasm distal to site of injection with absent pulse: radial, ulnar or both.
3. Delay in onset of anaesthesia.
4. Withdrawal of limb.

Management

1. Leave cannula in place.
2. Immediately inject:
   - Hydrocortisone 50 mg to inhibit the inflammatory response.
   - Papaverine 2 mg (dilute with 0.9% saline) for local vasodilatation.
   - Heparin 1000 U for local anti-thrombotic effect.
   - If there has been delay recognising the injury Streptokinase 1000 U/kg over 30 min. This may lyse any thrombus present.
3. Get help from a vascular surgeon.

4. Start an epoprostenol infusion intra-arterially at 1 ng/kg/min.
5. Sympathetic blockade of the limb (stellate ganglion or other appropriate sympathetic block of the affected side) may be considered.
6. Heparinise the patient (if no contraindications): 70–100 U/kg IV bolus, followed by 10–15 U/kg/h by continuous infusion, monitor KPTT.
7. Give parenteral opioid analgesia if required.
8. Nurse the affected limb at, or slightly above, heart level. It should not be dependent (below heart level) for prolonged periods.

MALIGNANT HYPERTHERMIA

Diagnosis

- Unexplained and unexpected tachycardia associated with an unexplained and unexpected increase in end-tidal CO_2.
- Masseter spasm after suxamethonium.

Immediate management

- Withdraw all trigger agents (anaesthetic vapours).
- Install clean anaesthetic breathing system and hyperventilate.
- Inform surgeon and abandon surgery, if feasible.
- Dantrolene 1 mg/kg IV and repeat if necessary up to 10 mg/kg.
- Measure core temperature, ABGs, potassium and CK.
- Surface cooling (tepid sponging to avoid skin vasoconstriction).

Intermediate management

- Control serious arrhythmias (β-blockers first line).
- Control hyperkalaemia and metabolic acidosis.

Later management

- Clotting screen to detect DIC.
- Take first voided urine sample for myoglobin estimation.
- Observe urine output for developing renal failure.
- Promote diuresis with fluids/mannitol.
- Repeat CK at 24 h.

Late management

- Consider other diagnosis and investigate as appropriate, e.g. thyroid function tests, WCC, CXR.

- Consider possibility of myopathy, neurological opinion, electromyography.
- Consider possibility of recreational drug injection (ecstasy).
- Consider possibility of neuroleptic malignant syndrome.
- Counsel patient and/or their family regarding implications of malignant hyperthermia.
- Refer patient to malignant hyperthermia unit.

Safe agents

- Thiopental
- Propofol
- Fentanyl
- Vecuronium
- Neostigmine
- Ketamine

- Etomidate
- Diazepam and midazolam
- Nitrous oxide
- Pancuronium
- Amide local anaesthetics

Avoid

- Suxamethonium
- All potent inhalational agents

Malignant Hyperthermia. Association of Anaesthetists in Great Britain and Ireland, London. 1998. www.aagbi.org/guidelines.html

NORMAL CARDIOVASCULAR VARIABLES AND THEIR CALCULATION

Variable	Formula	Normal range
Cardiac output (CO)	Heart rate × stroke volume	4–7 L/min
Cardiac index (CI)	CO/body surface area (BSA)	2.5–3.5 L/min/m²
Stroke volume (SV)	CO/HR × 1000	60–100 mL
Stroke volume index (SVI)	CI/HR × 1000	30–65 mL/m²
Systemic vascular resistance index (SVRI)	$MAP - CVP/CI \times 80$	1700–2600 dyne/s/cm⁵/m²
Pulmonary vascular resistance index (PVRI)	$MPAP - PCWP/CI \times 80$	45–225 dyne/s/cm⁵/m²
Left-ventricular stroke work index (LVSWI)	$SVI \times (MAP - PCWP) \times 0.0136$	43–61 g/m²
Right-ventricular stroke work index (RVSWI)	$SVI \times (MPAP - CVP) \times 0.0136$	7–12 g/m²
Arterial oxygen content (C_aO_2)	$Hb \times S_aO_2 \times 1.34/100$	18–20 mL/dL
Mixed venous oxygen content (C_vO_2)	$Hb \times S_vO_2 \times 1.34/100$	13–15 mL/dL
Oxygen extraction ratio (OER)	$C_aO_2 - C_vO_2/C_aO_2$	22–30%
Oxygen delivery index (DO_2I)	$CI \times C_aO_2 \times 10$	500–600 mL/min/m²
Oxygen consumption index (VO_2I)	$CI \times (C_aO_2 - C_vO_2) \times 10$	120–160 mL/min/m²
Pulmonary shunt fraction (Qs/Qt)	$C_cO_2 - C_aO_2/C_cO_2 - C_vO_2$	1–2%

HR, heart rate; MAP, mean arterial pressure; CVP, central venous pressure; MPAP, mean pulmonary arterial pressure; PCWP, pulmonary capillary wedge pressure; S_vO_2, mixed venous oxygen saturation; S_aO_2, arterial oxygen saturation; C_cO_2 oxygen content of ideal pulmonary end-capillary blood (usually assumed to be 100% for an $F_iO_2 > 0.21$).

Miller RD. *Anesthesia*, fifth edition. Churchill Livingston, Philadelphia, Pennsylvania, 2000

ANAESTHETIC INFORMATION

CHECKLIST FOR ANAESTHETIC APPARATUS

The following checks should be made before each operating session. The anaesthetist must be familiar with the equipment:

1. Check that the anaesthetic machine is connected to the electricity supply (if appropriate) and switched on:
   - Take note of any information or labelling on the anaesthetic machine referring to the current status of the machine. Particularly, attention should be paid to recent servicing. Servicing labels should be fixed in the service logbook.

2. Check that an oxygen analyser is present on the anaesthetic machine:
   - Ensure the analyser is switched on, checked and calibrated.
   - The oxygen sensor should be placed where it can monitor the composition of the gases leaving the common gas outlet.

3. Identify and take note of the gases that are being supplied by pipeline, confirming with a 'tug-test' that each pipeline is correctly inserted into appropriate gas supply terminal
   (*Note*: Carbon dioxide cylinders should not be present on the anaesthetic machine unless the anaesthetist intends to use it. A blanking plug should be fitted to any empty cylinder yoke):
   - Check that the anaesthetic machine is connected to a supply of oxygen and that an adequate supply of oxygen is available from a reserve oxygen cylinder.
   - Check that adequate supplies of other gases (nitrous oxide and air) are available and connected as appropriate. All cylinders should be securely seated and turned off after checking their contents.
   - Check that all pipeline pressure gauges in use on the anaesthetic machine indicates 400 kPa.

4. Check the operation of flowmeters:
   - Ensure that each control valve operates smoothly and that the bobbin moves freely throughout its range.
   - Check the operation of the emergency oxygen bypass control.

5. Check the vaporiser(s):
   - Ensure that each vaporiser is adequately but not overfilled and that the filling port is tightly closed.
   - Ensure that each vaporiser is correctly seated on the back bar and not tilted.

- Check the vaporiser for leaks (with vaporiser on and off) by temporarily occluding the common gas outlet with a flow of 5 L/min oxygen. There should be no leak from any of the vaporizer fitments and the flowmeter bobbin should dip.
- When checks have been completed turn the vaporisers off.
- A leak test should be performed immediately after changing any vaporiser.
- Removal of a vaporiser from a machine in order to refill it is not considered necessary.

6. Check the breathing system to be employed:
   - The system should be visually inspected for correct configuration. All connections should be secured by 'push and twist'.
   - A pressure leak test should be performed on the breathing system by occluding the patient port and compressing the reservoir bag.
   - The correct operation of unidirectional valves should be carefully checked.

7. Check that the ventilator is configured appropriately for its intended use:
   - Ensure that the ventilator tubing is correctly configured and securely attached.
   - Set the controls for use and ensure that an adequate pressure is generated during the inspiratory phase.
   - Check that the pressure relief valve functions.
   - Check that the disconnection alarm function correctly.
   - Ensure that an alternative means to ventilate the patient's lungs is available.

8. Check that anaesthetic gas-scavenging system is switched on and functioning correctly.
   - Ensure that the tubing is attached to the appropriate expiratory port(s) of the breathing system or ventilator.

9. Check that all ancillary equipment which may be needed is present and working:
   - This includes laryngoscopes, intubation forceps, bougies, etc. and appropriate sized face masks, airways, tracheal tubes and connectors.
   - Check that the suction apparatus is functioning and that all connections are secure.
   - Check that the patient can be tilted head-down on the trolley, operating table or bed.

10. Ensure that the appropriate monitoring equipment is present, switched on and calibrated ready for use:
    - Set all alarm limits as appropriate.

These checks are the responsibility of the anaesthetist and cannot be delegated.

Checklist for Anaesthetic Apparatus. Association of Anaesthetists of Great Britain and Ireland, London. 1997. www.aagbi.org/guidelines.html

MINIMAL MONITORING STANDARDS

There are recommended standards applied to all anaesthetics (except epidurals set up outside the operating theatre) administered by members of the department. They may be exceeded at any time as clinically appropriate.

All patients

The anaesthetist should be present throughout the conduct of the whole of a general anaesthetic, or a spinal or epidural anaesthetic until the patient is handed over to trained staff in a recovery room or ward area.
Exceptions:
- Briefly during radiation exposure.
- When the anaesthetist is urgently required in recovery or in an adjacent theatre, the care of a comprehensively monitored patient may be temporarily delegated to a trained assistant (non-anaesthetist doctor, ODP, or nurse).

Monitoring devices

The following monitoring devices are essential to the safe conduct of anaesthesia. If it is necessary to continue anaesthesia without a particular device, the anaesthetist must clearly record the reasons for this in the anaesthetic record.

Induction of anaesthesia

- Pulse oximeter
- Non-invasive blood pressure monitor
- Electrocardiograph
- Capnograph

The following must also be available:

- A nerve stimulator whenever a muscle relaxant is used
- A means of measuring the patient's temperature

Maintenance of anaesthesia

- The same used for induction
- Vapour analyser

Recovery

- Pulse oximeter
- Non-invasive blood pressure

The following must be immediately available:

- Electrocardiograph
- Nerve stimulator
- Means of measuring temperature
- Capnograph

(See also checklist for anaesthetic apparatus.)

Recommendations for Standards of Monitoring during Anaesthesia and Recovery. Association of Anaesthetists of Great Britain and Ireland, London. 2000. www.aagbi.org/guidelines.html

MAPLESON CIRCUITS

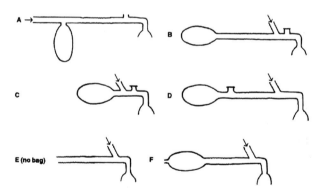

A: Magill and Lack; B: Mapleson B; C: Mapelson C; D: Bain; E: Ayres T piece; F: Ayres T piece with Jackson Rees modification (the arrows indicate entry of fresh gas to the system). Bain co-axial modification: fresh gas tube inside breathing tube.

Fresh gas flow required for the Mapleson circuits:

Circuit	Spontaneous breathing	IPPV
Magill and Lack	MV × 1	MV × 2+
Mapleson B	MV × 2	MV × 2–2½
Mapleson C	MV × 2	MV × 2–2½
Bain circuit	MV × 2–3	MV × 1–2
Ayres T piece	MV × 2–3	MV × 3
Jackson Rees	MV × 2–3	MV × 2

MV, minute ventilation (70 mL/kg/min)

MAC VALUES FOR ADULTS AND PAEDIATRIC PATIENTS

Inhalational agent	MAC% (in air/O_2)	
	In children	In adults
Nitrous oxide		105
Halothane	0.87	0.75
Enflurane		1.7
Isoflurane	1.3–1.6	1.2
Sevoflurane	2.5	2.0
Desflurane	7–8	6.0

MAC, minimum alveolar concentration

The addition of nitrous oxide decreases the requirements of other volatile agents – 65% nitrous oxide, decreases the MAC of the inhalational anaesthetic by approximately 50%.

Aitkenhead AR, Rowbotham DJ and Smith G. *Textbook of Anaesthesia,* fourth edition. Churchill Livingstone, London. 2001

Morgan GE, Mikkhail MS and Murray MJ. *Clinical Anesthesiology*, third edition. International Edition. 2002

GUIDE TO LARYNGEAL MASK AIRWAY (LMA) AND TRACHEAL TUBE SIZES

Formulae for tube sizes and lengths

$$\text{Tube size (mm)} = \frac{\text{age (years)}}{4} + 4.0$$

$$\text{Oral length (cm)} = \frac{\text{age (years)}}{2} + 12$$

$$\text{Nasal length (cm)} = \frac{\text{age (years)}}{2} + 15$$

Guide to tracheal tube sizes

Age	Tube size (mm)	Oral length (cm)*
Premature	2.5	10
Newborn	3.0	11
1–6 months	3.5	11
6–12 months	4.0	12
2 years	4.5	13
4 years	5.0	14
6 years	5.5	15–16
8 years	6.0	16–17
10 years	6.5	17–18
12 years	7.0	18–22
≥14 years		
Females	7.0	20–24
Males	8.0	

* Add 2–3 cm for nasal tubes

Miller RD. *Anesthesia,* fifth edition. 2000

Below 8 years of age an uncuffed tracheal tube should be used.

Guide to laryngeal mask airway (LMA) sizes

Size of LMA	Suggested weight of patient (kg)	Maximum cuff inflation volume (mL)
1	<5	4
1.5	5–10	7
2	10–20	10
2.5	20–30	14
3	Children/small adults >30 kg	20
4	Normal and large adults	30
5	Large adults	40

Miller RD. *Anesthesia,* fifth edition. 2000

ADULT ANAESTHETIC AND RELATED DRUG DOSES

Drug	Dose/kg	Average adult dose*
Premedications		
Diazepam		5 mg O
Lorazepam		2–3 mg O
Midazolam		2.5–7.5 mg IM
Temazepam		20–40 mg O
Pethidine	1 mg/kg	25–100 mg IM
Promethazine		25–50 mg O
IV induction agents		
Etomidate	300 µg/kg	10 mg IV
Ketamine	8 mg/kg IM	500 mg IM
	1–2 mg/kg IV	150 mg IV
Propofol	1.5–2.5 mg/kg	100–175 mg IV
	4–12 mg/kg/h infusion	
Thiopental	3–7 mg/kg	200–500 mg IV
Analgesics		
Alfentanil	15–50 µg/kg	0.25–1 mg IV
Buprenorphine		200–400 µg SL
		300–600 µg IM
Diamorphine		2.5 mg IV
		5 mg IM
Fentanyl	1–3 µg/kg	50–100 µg IV
Morphine	0.2 mg/kg IM	10–15 mg IM
	0.025–0.05 mg/kg IV	2–5 mg IV
Pethidine	0.5–2 mg/kg IM	50–100 mg IM
	0.3–0.5 mg/kg IV	25–50 mg IV
Remifentanil anaesthesia	0.5–1 µg/kg/min induction	
	0.05–1 µg/kg/min maintenance	
Sedation ICU	6–45 µg/kg/h	
Anti-emetics		
Cyclizine		50 mg IV/IM/O
Metoclopramide		10 mg IV/IM/O
Ondansetron		4 mg IV/IM/O
Perphenazine		4 mg IM
Prochlorperazine		12.5 mg IM
		5 mg O

Continued

ADULT ANAESTHETIC AND RELATED DRUG DOSES (continued)

Drug	Dose/kg	Average adult dose*
Muscle relaxants (incremental doses in brackets)		
Atracurium		
Bolus	300–600 µg/kg	25–50 mg IV
	(100–200 µg/kg)	
Infusion	300–600 µg/kg/h	20–40 mg/h
Cis-atrcurium	150 µg/kg	10 mg IV
	(30 µg/kg)	(2 mg)
Mivacurium	70–250 µg/kg	7–10 mg IV
	(100 µg/kg)	(5–10 mg)
Pancuronium	50–100 µg/kg	4–8 mg IV
	(10–20 µg/kg)	(1–2 mg)
Rocuronium	600 µg/kg	30–50 mg IV
	(150 µg/kg)	(10–15 mg)
Suxamethonium	1 mg/kg	75–100 mg IV
Vecuronium	80–100 µg/kg	4–8 mg IV
	(20–30 µg/kg)	(1.5–2.5 mg)
Anticholinergic drugs		
Atropine	0.01 mg/kg	0.3–0.6 mg IV
reversal	0.01–0.02 mg/kg	0.6–1.2 mg
Glycopyrronium	4–5 µg/kg	200–400 µg IV
reversal	10–15 µg/kg	400–600 µg
Hysocine		0.2–0.6 mg IM
Anticholinesterase drugs		
Edrophonium		10 mg IV
Neostigmine	30–50 µg/kg	2.5–5 mg IV
Reversal – opioids		
Naloxone	1.5–3 µg/kg	100–200 µg IV
		100 µg every 2 min
		as required
Reversal – benzodiazepines		
Flumazenil**		200 µg initial dose
		100 µg every 30 s to
		a maximum of 1 mg

* The doses given in this table are for fit young patients. Doses will need adjustment in the elderly or ill patients
** Do not use in mixed drug overdose/head injuries

SL, sublingual

BNF 43, March 2002. www.bnf.org

LOCAL ANAESTHETIC MAXIMUM SAFE DOSES FOR REGIONAL ANALGESIA

Drug	Maximum dose (mg/kg)
Bupivacaine	2
Lidocaine (plain)	4.5
Lidocaine with epinephrine	7
Prilocaine	8

LOCAL ANAESTHETIC BLOCKS: DRUG DOSES

Block	Drug	Dose
Retrobulbar eye	Lidocaine 2% or Prilocaine 2%	1.2–2 mL complete akinesia: 4 mL
Stellate ganglion	Lidocaine 1% or Bupivacaine 0.5%	10 mL
Upper limb		
Brachial plexus		
Interscalene	Lidocaine 1%,	
Supraclavicular	Bupivacaine 0.25–0.5% or	20–40 mL
Axillary	Levobupivacaine 0.25–0.5%	
IV regional	Prilocaine 0.5–1%	40 mL
Lateral cutaneous		3.5 mL
Ulnar	Lidocaine 1%,	5 mL
Median	Bupivacaine 0.5% or	5 mL
Radial	Levobupivacaine 0.25–0.5%	5–10 mL
Lower limb		
Femoral		10–20 mL
Lateral cutaneous nerve	Lidocaine 1%,	6 mL
'3-in-1' block	Bupivacaine 0.5% or	20–30 mL
Sciatic	Levobupivacaine 0.5%	20 mL
Ankle blocks		
Tibial, sural, saphenous, superficial and deep peroneal nerves	Lidocaine 1%	5–10 mL
Intercostal	Bupivacaine 0.5%	3 mL per rib

Continued

LOCAL ANAESTHETIC BLOCKS: DRUG DOSES (continued)

Block	Drug	Dose
Spinal		
Saddle	Hyperbaric bupivacaine 0.5% or	1 mL
Lumbo-thoracic	Levobupivacaine 0.5%	2–3 mL
Epidural		
Lumbar	Bupivacaine 0.5% or	
	Levobupivacaine 0.5–0.75%	10–20 mL
Obstetrics		
Analgesia	Bupivacaine 0.25% or	
	Levobupivacaine 0.25%	8–10 mL
Caesarean	Bupivacaine 0.5% or	
	Levobupivacaine 0.5%	15–30 mL
Thoracic	Bupivacaine 0.25%–0.5%	2.5–8 mL
Caudal (adults)	Bupivacaine 0.5% or Lidocaine 1%	20 mL
Continuous	Bupivacaine 0.1% +	4–8 mL/h
infusion	Fentanyl 2 μg/mL	

DERMATOME CHART

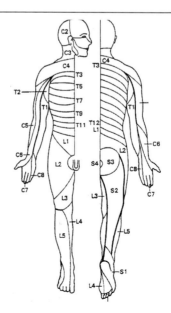

PAEDIATRIC ANAESTHETIC INFORMATION

PAEDIATRIC ANAESTHETIC AND RELATED DRUG DOSES

Premedication
- Requirements depend on patient and surgery
- Avoid IM injections, if possible
- Infants below 5 kg – avoid sedatives
- EMLA/Ametop (Tetracaine/Amethocaine) routinely (NB: Be careful with EMLA in small infants, prilocaine may cause methaemoglobinemia)
- Anticholinergic drugs may be given pre-operatively to prevent reflex bradycardia and reduce airway secretions

Atropine	0.02 mg/kg IM; 0.04 mg/kg O
Midazolam (>10 kg)	0.5 mg/kg O
Temazepam (older children)	0.5 mg/kg O
Triclofos (5–10 kg)	50–75 mg/kg O
Trimeprazine (Vallergan®)	2–3 mg/kg O
Hyoscine	0.01 mg/kg (maximum 0.4 mg) IM
Pethidine	0.06–0.08 mL/kg (1.5–2 mg/kg) IM

IV induction agents
Etomidate	0.3 mg/kg IV
Ketamine	2 mg/kg IV (5–10 mg/kg IM)
Propofol	2–3 mg/kg IV (over 3 years of age only)
Thiopental	4–6 mg/kg IV (neonates 2 mg/kg)

Muscle relaxants (incremental doses in brackets)
Atracurium	
Bolus	0.5 mg/kg (0.25 mg/kg) IV
Infusion	8 µg/kg/min
Cis-atracurium	0.1–0.4 mg/kg (0.05 mg/kg) IV
Mivacurium	
Bolus	0.1–0.2 mg/kg (0.1 mg/kg) IV
Infusion	10–15 µg/kg/min
Pancuronium	
Infants and children	0.1 mg/kg IV
Neonates	0.06 mg/kg IV
Rocuronium	0.6 mg/kg (0.1–0.2 mg/kg) IV

Continued

PAEDIATRIC ANAESTHETIC AND RELATED DRUG DOSES *(continued)*

Suxamethonium intubation	1–2 mg/kg IV
Vecuronium	
Bolus	0.1 mg/kg IV
Infusion	1.5–2 μg/kg/min

Reversal

Atropine	0.02 mg/kg IV
Glycopyrronium	10–20 μg/kg IV
Neostigmine	50 μg/kg IV

Analgesics (intra-operative)

Alfentanil	30–50 μg/kg IV
Codeine	1–1.5 mg/kg IM
Fentanyl	2–5 μg/kg IV
Morphine	50–200 μg/kg IM
Pethidine	1 mg/kg IM
Remifentanil	
Bolus	0.5–1 μg/kg IV
Infusion	0.05–1 μg/kg/min IV

Analgesics (post-operative)

Analgesia is given with caution in the neonate after individual assessment
    <8 kg: seek advice
    >8 kg: safe if child is normal

Codeine	1 mg/kg 4–6-hourly IM/O/PR
Fentanyl	4 μg/kg/min IV infusion
Morphine	0.2 mg/kg IM/IV
Paracetamol	15 mg/kg 4–6-hourly O
	20 mg/kg 6-hourly PR
Diclofenac (>6 months)	1–3 mg/kg/day in divided doses
	8-hourly O/PR
	50 mg dispersible tablets available
Ibuprofen (>7 kg)	7–10 mg/kg 8-hourly O

Sedatives

Baclofen	5–15 mg O
Chloral hydrate	30 mg/kg O
Diazepam	100–200 μg/kg IV
Midazolam	20 μg/kg IV
Phenobarbitone	1–2 mg/kg IV to control seizures

Continued

Promethazine	0.5–1 mg/kg O
Triclofos elixir	30 mg/kg O

Antibiotics

Amikacin	8 mg/kg 12-hourly IV/IM
Amoxycillin	25 mg/kg 6-hourly IV/IM
Ampicillin	up to 50 mg/kg 6-hourly for severe infections IV/IM
Benzylpenicillin	25–50 mg/kg 6-hourly IV/IM
Cefotaxime	30 mg/kg 8-hourly IV/IM*
Cefuroxime	25 mg/kg 6-hourly IV/IM*
Erythromycin	6–12 mg/kg 6-hourly IV infusion**
Flucloxacillin	
<2 years	62.5–125 mg 6-hourly IV/IM
>2 years	125–250 mg 6-hourly IV/IM
Gentamicin	2 mg/kg 8-hourly IV*
Metronidazole	7.5 mg/kg 8-hourly IV infusion
Meropenem	10–40 mg/kg 8-hourly IV
Tobramycin	2.0 mg/kg 8-hourly IV*
Vancomycin	20 mg/kg 12-hourly IV infusion over 1 h*

Others

Adenosine	30–40 μg/kg IV
Aminophylline	
Bolus	5 mg/kg IV
Infusion	0.8 mg/kg/h*
Cimetidine	5–10 mg/kg 6-hourly O*
Dexamethasone	0.25 mg/kg IV
Flumazenil	
Bolus	1–2 μg/kg IV
Infusion	1–5 μg/kg/h
Furosemide	1.0 mg/kg IV
Hydrocortisone	
<1 year	25 mg 6–8-hourly IV/IM
1–5 years	50 mg 6–8-hourly IV/IM
6–12 years	100 mg 6–8-hourly IV/IM
Lidocaine	1 mg/kg IV
Metoclopramide	0.015 mg/kg IV/IM/O 8-hourly
Naloxone	1.5–3 μg/kg IV repeat every 3–5 min as required
	0.5 μg/kg IV for itching, urinary retention

Continued

PAEDIATRIC ANAESTHETIC INFORMATION 34

PAEDIATRIC ANAESTHETIC AND RELATED DRUG DOSES (continued)

Salbutamol
<18 months	1.5–2.5 mg 6-hourly nebulised
>18 months	2.5 mg nebulised 6-hourly

*Dose adjustment necessary in renal failure
**Dose adjustment necessary in hepatic failure

Sumner E and Hatch DJ. *Paediatric Anaesthesia,* second edition. Arnold publishers, London. 2002.

BNF 43, March 2002. www.bnf.org

USEFUL PAEDIATRIC INFORMATION

Blood volume

Newborn to 10 kg	85 mL/kg
10–20 kg	80 mL/kg
20–30 kg	75 mL/kg
30–40 kg	70 mL/kg
>40 kg	65 mL/kg

Basal fluid requirements
4 mL/kg/h for the first 10 kg body weight
2 mL/kg/h for the second 10 kg body weight
1 mL/kg/h for weight over 20 kg

Electrolyte requirements

Sodium	2 mmol/kg/day
Potassium	2 mmol/kg/day
Calcium	1 mmol/kg/day

Normal ventilation values at rest

Weight (kg)	Minute volume (mL)	Tidal volume (mL)	Frequency (breaths/min)
2	480	14–16	30–45
3	600	17–25	25–40
10	1680	80	21
20	3040	160	19
30	4000	250	17
40	4800	320	15
50	5200	400	12

INTENSIVE CARE INFORMATION AND DATA

SOME ASPECTS OF VENTILATORY SUPPORT

Oxygen face masks

Low-flow systems

These include nasal canulae and simple low-volume oxygen masks. The F_iO_2 they supply is variable depending on the oxygen flow and the minute ventilation of the patient.

High-flow systems

These use the high pressure of the oxygen supply to entrain air through a Venturi system. This leads to an increase in fresh gas flow. The degree of air entrainment allows a predictable F_iO_2 to be given. The high flow usually meets the peak inspiratory flow rate resulting in a known F_iO_2, independent of the patient's ventilation. An alternative system has a reservoir bag that stores the fresh gas. It can give a high oxygen concentration, but this is dependent on the rate and depth of the patients breathing.

Routine for establishing mechanical ventilation

1. Establish an IV line and appropriate monitoring. Insert a tracheal tube (obtain help with this if you are not proficient with tracheal intubation).
2. In adults, set the ventilator to deliver about 4–6 mL/kg tidal volume,* at a respiratory rate of 12 breaths/min. Avoid excessive airway pressure (plateau pressure 30 cmH$_2$O).
3. Apply 5 cm PEEP, if indicated (not if the patient is wheezy).
4. Set the F_iO_2 to 0.2 above that which the patient was breathing before artificial ventilaton (if the P_aO_2 was adequate).
5. Look at the chest to ensure that it is moving.
6. Listen to the chest to ensure bilateral air entry.
7. Measure the ABGs. Aim for a P_aO_2 of between 8 and 10 kPa and a P_aCO_2 in the normal range. If the P_aO_2 is too high, decrease the F_iO_2; if the P_aO_2 is too low, increase the F_iO_2; if the P_aCO_2 is too high, increase the minute volume (usually by increasing the frequency); if the P_aCO_2 is too low, decrease the minute ventilation. In some patients, a

high P_aCO_2 is accepted (e.g. asthmatics). Low levels of P_aCO_2 should only be used as an adjunct to reduce brain volume during craniotomy and should be allowed to increase once the retractors are removed.

8. Obtain a CXR to confirm correct placement of the tracheal tube.
9. Recheck the ABGs until satisfactory P_aO_2 and P_aCO_2 are obtained. Try to keep the F_iO_2 below 0.6 to avoid the risk of oxygen toxicity. If necessary increase the PEEP.

* Brower RG, Matthay MA, Morris A, Schoenfeld D, Thompson BT and Wheeler A. Ventilation of lower tidal volumes as compared with traditional tidal volumes for acute lung injury and the acute respiratory distress syndrome. *New Engl J Med* 2000; **342**: 1301–8.

PEEP/CPAP

Continuous positive airway pressure (CPAP) during spontaneous ventilation and positive end-expiratory pressure (PEEP) during artificial ventilation can be used to re-expand collapsed areas of lung and therefore reduce ventilation/perfusion mismatch. Excessive levels can be detrimental causing barotrauma and a decrease in cardiac output. They should not be used in patients with obstructive airways disease/asthma.

MICROBIOLOGY

Suggested initial antibiotic regimens

These regimens are for empirical treatment before culture results are known. The doses are for patients with normal renal and hepatic function. Whenever possible, seek expert advice from a microbiologist. The recommendations are based on the common antibiotic sensitivities of the bacteria found in our patients. These sensitivities vary from ICU to ICU.

Septic shock (including abdominal sepsis)
  Cefotaxime 1–2 g IV 8-hourly + Metronidazole 500 mg IV 8-hourly

IV line infection
  Vancomycin 1 g IV infusion, assay after 12 h

Community-acquired pneumonia
  Cefotaxime 2 g IV 8-hourly (1 g when symptoms are improving) + Erythromycin 1 g IV 6-hourly

Aspirative pneumonia
   Cefotaxime 2 g IV 8-hourly + Metronidazole 500 mg IV 8-hourly
   for 3 days, then 12-hourly
Ventilator-acquired pneumonia
   Meropenem 1 g 6–8 hourly
   Vancomycin 1 g daily (if MRSA endemic)

Meningitis
   Cefotaxime 2 g IV 6-hourly – consult a microbiologist after the first dose

---

Antibiotic doses in renal and hepatic failure

Drug	Normal renal function	CrCl 20–50 mL/min	CrCl 10–20 mL/min	CrCl <10 mL/min or dialysis	Liver failure
Cefotaxime	1 g 8-hourly	1 g 8-hourly	1 g 8-hourly	0.5–1 g 8–12-hourly	
Ceftazidime	1 g 8-hourly	1 g 12-hourly	1 g daily	500 mg daily	
Erythromicin	1 g 6-hourly	1 g 6-hourly	1 g 6-hourly	500 mg 8-hourly	500 mg 6-hourly
Gentamicin	5 mg/kg daily	According to serum levels			
Metronidazole	500 mg 8-hourly			500 mg 12-hourly	
Vancomycin	1 g 12-hourly	According to serum levels			

Gentamicin

- 5 mg/kg daily (round to the nearest 40 mg) as a once-only dose.
- Measure baseline renal function before starting gentamicin.
- Take a pre-dose (trough) blood sample before the second dose and every 2nd or 3rd day, more frequently if renal function is changing or levels are abnormal.
- Avoid giving gentamicin for more than 5 days whenever possible.

Gentamicin serum levels (at 24h)

Pre-dose	<1 mg/L	Satisfactory
	1–2 mg/L	Borderline (reduce dose frequency to 36-hourly)
	>2 mg/L	Unsatisfactory (change to alternative agent if possible or discuss use of lower dose regimen with microbiologist)

Vancomycin serum levels

Renal function	Perform vancomycin levels
Normal (CrCl > 50 mL/min)	Pre- and 1 h post-third dose, then twice weekly
CrCl 10–50 mL/min	Pre-and 1 h post-third dose, then thrice weekly
CrCl < 10 mL/min or haemodialysis/CVVHD	Daily single, timed serum level

Recommended vancomycin levels

Pre-dose	5–10 mg/mL
Post-dose	20–40 mg/mL

Once patients are established on a regimen with a satisfactory pre- and post-dose serum levels, it may be sufficient to assay the pre-dose level only. Discuss this with a microbiologist.

A Guide to Antibiotic Therapy in Adult Patients. Addenbrooke's Hospital NHS Trust. December 2001

MANAGING PYREXIA OF UNKNOWN ORIGIN IN THE CRITICALLY ILL PATIENT

Examination

Full clinical examination carried out with particular attention paid to

- chest (chest infection),
- heart (subacute bacterial endocarditis),
- ears (acute otitis media),
- mouth (dental abscess),
- abdomen (abscess),
- line sites.

Investigation

- FBC with white cell count and differential.
- Specimens to microbiology, blood cultures (several), urine, wound swab, CVP line tips, sputum, bronchial lavage.
- Specimens to virology (remember respiratory serology). Two specimens of serum, taken over 10 days.

- CXR.
- Echocardiogram (subacute bacterial endocarditis).
- Ultrasound or CT of abdomen (subphrenic or other abscess).
- White cell scan.
- CT scan chest.

OLIGURIA AND ANURIA

Acute renal failure is usually associated with oliguria, not anuria.

Anuria follows – catheter in the wrong orifice or blocked, inadvertant tying of the ureters at operation and vascular accident.

Investigation

1. Review the patient's fluid and electrolyte balance.
2. Review the drug chart and confirm that no nephrotoxic drugs are being given; if aminoglycosides or the nephrotoxic drugs are being used, ensure the plasma levels are not in the toxic range.
3. Measure the plasma urea, electrolytes and osmolality.
4. Measure the urinary electrolytes and urine osmolality.
5. Ultrasound the kidneys to see if there is an acute, obstructive uropathy.

Treatment

Pre-renal failure

Give a volume expander, or fluid appropriate to replace the losses.

Renal failure

- Ensure that pre-renal and obstructive causes have been excluded.
- Give furosemide 20 mg, and 1 h later if there is no response, give a further 80 mg of furosemide.
- If there is no response to furosemide, give mannitol (1 g/kg IV) over 1 h. Mannitol produces an increase in intravascular volume, and care is necessary, if the patient is at risk of pulmonary oedema.
- If there is no response, give furosemide (250 mg IV) over 1 h.
- When a diuresis starts either because of treatment or recovery from acute renal failure, tubular function is impaired and sodium conservation is impaired. Measure the urinary sodium and use an appropriate replacement fluid.

- If diuresis with furosemide or mannitol is transient, it may be maintained with an infusion of mannitol (1.5–2 g/kg/24 h) or furosemide (5–10 mg/h).
- If there is no response to these measures, restrict the total fluid input to the urine output plus an allowance for insensible loss. Do not restrict the nitrogen intake, start renal support so adequate nutrition can be given.

Renal support may be necessary when renal function is inadequate. Three methods are available: haemodialysis, peritoneal dialysis and continuous haemodiafiltration with or without dialysis.

Obstructive uropathy

This is treated by ureteric or urethral catheterisation, or percutaneous drainage of the renal pelvis.

MANAGEMENT OF HYPERKALAEMIA

Aim to reduce plasma potassium towards the safe range and reverse cardiac manifestations. If plasma potassium is above 5.5 mmol/L, stop drugs that could contribute to hyperkalaemia and review potassium intakes in feeds and infusions. If plasma potassium is above 6.5 mmol/L:

- *Calcium:* 5–10 mL of 10% calcium gluconate given rapidly, repeated where necessary up to 30 mL or 3–5 mL of 10% calcium chloride, for patients with severe hyperkalaemia or life-threatening dysrhythmias. Its effect is rapid but short lived.
- *Sodium bicarbonate:* 50 mL of 8.4% solution IV in normovolaemic patients with metabolic acidosis will promote cellular uptake of potassium and decrease plasma potassium within 15 min. In the hypovolaemic acidotic patient, acidosis should be treated with appropriate volume replacement.
- *Glucose insulin infusion:* 15 U of insulin in 50 mL 50% glucose given centrally over 60 min, and 15–20 units of insulin in 500 mL 10–20% glucose over 30–60 min, promotes cellular uptake of potassium. It takes up to 1 h for peak effect, and may be repeated 3–6 h later. It is usually inadequate in hypercatabolic patients and those with established renal failure.
- *Furosemide:* furosemide in patients with some renal function will increase potassium excretion.
- *Cation-exchange resins:* these are useful in patients with isolated renal failure. In the critically ill patient where gut function varies, haemodyalisis or haemofiltration is a better choice.

Haemofiltration and/or hemodialyis should be used in patients where the previous methods fail and in those with acute or acute-on-chronic renal failure.

Before giving the patient any drugs try and find out what is causing the discomfort. Try correcting these causes before giving drugs, e.g.:

- Are they frightened? Will talking to them remove their fear?
- Is the ventilator set properly for them?
- Do they have a full bowel or bladder?
- Does the plaster cast itch?
- To help them sleep do they need a quiet side room, eyeshades and earplugs?

The next step is to relive any pain they may be suffering from surgical incisions, broken bones, pleurisy, pericarditis, etc. If the patient needs mechanical ventilation, give opioids. Remifentanil (6–15 μg/kg/h by infusion), morphine (2 mg bolus doses until the pain is controlled or 5–20 mg/h), fentanyl (50 μg bolus doses or 100–200 μg/h by infusion). Discomfort caused by the tracheal tube and/or the ventilator can also be treated using opioids at the same doses.

Relief of pain may be all that 50% of patients who are receiving mechanical ventilation need. However, in the other half, a benzodiazepine may be useful to relieve anxiety (midazolam 1–2 mg bolus doses or 1–5 mg/h by infusion). Alternatively, if the patient wants to be sleepier, then a hypnotic agent such as propofol (50–100 mg/h) can be used.

If the patient is unconscious, then sedative and analgesic agents should be stopped each day and the patient is allowed to recover. If this takes a long time, then consider smaller doses of the drug or give the drug by bolus rather than infusion or use a different drug. Do not use a routine wake-up tests, if the patient needs an $F_IO_2 > 0.85$ or has raised intracranial pressure.

Use a sedation score (see page 51). This will ensure that the proper attention is given to the safe use of the drugs.

Dexmedetomidine (currently unavailable in Europe) may be given in patients needing short-term mechanical ventilation after operation to relive post-operative pain and anxiolysis beyond extubation. Loading dose is 0.3–0.5 μg/kg over 20 min and infusion 0.2–0.7 μg/kg/h. Dexmedetomidine can cause hypertension associated to bradycardia due to an α_2-agonism effect.

Withdrawal may occur when any sedative or analgesic drug has been given. A gradual withdrawal or a change to another agent may overcome this. Alternatively, clonidine (4 μg/kg over 30–60 min loading dose, and 0.25–0.75 μg/kg/h infusion) or haloperidol (2.5 mg bolus doses to a maximum of 20 mg) may be useful.

If the patient is conscious and not needing mechanical ventilation, then a patient-controlled analgesia system giving 1 mg doses of morphine on demand, with a lock-out time of 5 min may work well. In some patients, regional analgesia using an epidural or intercostal nerve blocks may give excellent analgesia for thoracic or abdominal trauma or surgery. Peripheral nerve blocks may be useful for some limb trauma. Besides giving the best possible analgesia, regional techniques avoid respiratory depression caused by opioids.

NUTRITION

Where possible, feed patients enterally; otherwise nutrition can be given parenterally, either via a peripheral (low-osmolarity solutions) or central vein. Peripheral feeds are associated with a higher incidence of thrombophlebitis and provide limited concentrations of carbohydrate and amino acids. In intensive care, total parenteral nutrition is usually given through a central line.

Energy requirements

The total calorie intake should be approximately equivalent to normal resting energy requirements, i.e. 25–30 kcal/kg/day, as a mixture of carbohydrate and fat.

Carbohydrate

One gram of carbohydrate supplies 4 cal. This is supplied in solutions of 10%, 20%, 40% or 50% glucose. Nutrition is usually started with 200 g glucose (1 L 20% glucose) in 24 h. If blood glucose is >6.0 mmol/L, start insulin infusion: 50 U of insulin in 50 mL of 0.9% saline. If little or no insulin is required 400 g and then 500 g glucose could be given over the following two 24-h periods. If insulin requirements are high (>6 U/h), do not increase the glucose concentration.

Insulin-sliding scale suitable for an adult

Blood glucose (mmol/L)	Insulin infusion rate (U/h)
6–7.9	1
8–9.9	2
10–12	3
>12	4

Aim to keep blood glucose level between 4.5 and 6.0 mmol/L

If blood glucose <3.0 mmol/L: 50 mL of 50% glucose IV bolus; stop insulin infusion

Lipid solutions

One gram of fat supplies 9 cal. Intralipid is one fat source, available as 10% and 20% solutions. Caution is necessary in patients who are:

- deeply jaundiced,
- severely hypoxaemic,
- thrombocytopaenic.

Start with 1–2 days of 500 mL 10% intralipid over 24 h. This may be increased to 20% depending on individual patient requirement. If lipaemia is detected, increase the duration of administration or decrease the daily dose.

Reduce the amount of lipid solution, if the patient is being given propofol for sedation. Propofol is dissolved in lipid.

Nitrogen requirements

One gram nitrogen equals 6.25 g protein which is equal to 25 g wet muscle. Nitrogen requirements vary greatly. The correct amount to administer can be derived from tables or from measurement of urinary urea. However, usually patients need 14 g nitrogen per day. All of the commonly available amino acid solutions contain sufficient essential amino acids.

Vitamin requirements

Most water-soluble vitamin preparations contain sufficient quantities of all vitamins. However, some require additional B_{12} and folic acid. Give folic acid 15 mg/day and B_{12} 1 mg monthly.

There are body stores of lipid-soluble vitamins and replacement is not needed as frequently. Vitlipid can be given dissolved in intralipid on alternate days.

Daily administration of proprietary water-soluble vitamin preparations may be needed.

Phosphate

Glucose and insulin feeding results in a large decrease in plasma phosphate. Hypophosphataemia can be prevented by the administration of potassium or sodium hydrogen phosphate 20–30 mmol/day.

Laboratory monitoring

1. Daily Hb, WCC, plasma urea and electrolytes when the patient is seriously ill – may be reduced during recovery (other problems permitting); blood sugar may need frequent monitoring initially.
2. Three times a week liver function tests, plasma protein and albumin, calcium and phosphate.
3. Once weekly magnesium.

Big-bag nutrition

The total requirements for parenteral nutrition for 24 h can be mixed in a 2–3-L bag. This is easy, more accurate and has a smaller risk of infection but may lack the flexibility needed in the management of the seriously ill patient.

Different formulations are available for patients with specific fluid, electrolyte or nutritional needs, e.g. renal failure.

It is tempting to overfeed patients, this should be resisted as it has many complications.

Specific considerations

Renal failure: is accompanied by intolerance to fluids and an increase in the plasma levels of K^+, Mg^{++} and phosphate. Frequent monitoring of these analytes is needed and the amounts administered reduced to maintain appropriate plasma levels.

Liver failure: most patients will have increased losses of K^+, Mg^{++}, Zn and may be treated with fluid restriction for the presence of ascites. Encephalopathy frequently accompanies liver failure. Some protein should be provided during this time.

Respiratory failure: most patients with isolated respiratory failure can be treated by applying the general principles for nutrition support.

HALF-LIVES AND TIMES TO REACH STEADY STATE OF COMMONLY USED DRUGS IN THE CRITICALLY ILL

Some drugs have serum concentrations measured to guide dosage. The table in page 46 shows the half-life and time to steady state. There is usually, little value in measuring serum concentrations more frequently than time to steady state.

Drug	Ideal sampling time (sample)	Average plasma half-life (h)	Time to steady state (days)	Therapeutic range
Amiodarone	Pre-dose (serum)	240–2400	60–90	0.5–2.0 mg/L
Carbamazepine (Tegretol®)	Pre-dose (serum)	36	7	30–50 μmol/L
Cyclosporin (Sandimmun®)	Just before morning dose (whole blood) in an EDTA tube	8–20	2–4	Depends on clinical indication and may change with time
Digoxin (Lanoxin®, etc.)	6–8 h post-dose (serum)	36	7	1.0–2.6 nmol/L, >3.8 nmol/L toxicity inevitable
Ethosuximide (Zarontin®)	Pre-dose (serum)	50	10	280–700 μmol/L
Phenobarbitone (Luminal®, etc.)	Pre-dose (serum)	67 (children) 96 (adult)	12 (children) 20 (adults)	50–100 μmol/L (neonate) 40–170 μmol/L (child/adult)
Phenytoin (Epanutin®)	Pre-dose (serum)	13–46	14	40–80 μmol/L
Primidone (Mysoline®)	Pre-dose (serum)	8	2	25–70 μmol/L
Theophylline (including that released from aminophylline)	Pre-dose (serum)	24 (neonates) 4 (children) 9 (non-smoking adults) 4 (smokers)	5 (neonates) 1–2 (children) 2 (non-smoking adults) 1–2 (smokers)	55–110 μmol/L (adult) >190 μmol/L high risk of cardiac arrythmias
Valproate (Epilim®)	Pre-dose (serum)	12	3	400–600 μmol/L

BRAIN DEATH

Criteria used for the diagnosis of brainstem death are given below.

Preconditions

- The patient is in apnoeic coma (i.e. unresponsive and on a ventilator, with no spontaneous respiratory efforts).
- Irremediable structural brain damage due to a disorder that can cause brainstem death has been diagnosed with certainty (e.g. head injury, intracranial haemorrhage).

Exclusions

- The possibility that unresponsive apnoea is the result of poisons, sedative drugs, or neuromuscular-blocking agents must be excluded. Blood and urine should be tested for the presence of drugs, if there is any doubt.
- Hypothermia must be excluded as a cause of coma. Central body temperature should be >35°C.
- There must be no significant metabolic or endocrine disturbance that could produce or contribute to coma or cause it to persist. There should be no profound abnormality of the plasma electrolytes, acid–base balance, or blood glucose levels.

Assessment of brainstem function

- Confirm the absence of oculocephalic reflexes.
- The pupils should be fixed and unresponsive to bright light. Both direct and consensual light reflexes should be examined.
- Corneal reflexes should be absent.
- Vestibulo-ocular reflexes should be absent ('caloric testing'). Remember that gentamicin can cause end-organ poisoning, and central pathways may be impaired by drugs. Ensure that the ears are clear of wax.
- There must be no motor responses within the cranial nerve territory to painful stimuli applied centrally or peripherally. Spinal reflexes may be present.
- There must be no gag or cough reflexes in response to pharyngeal, laryngeal or tracheal stimulation.
- Spontaneous respiration should be absent. ABGs should be taken to confirm $P_aCO_2 > 6.7$ kPa, 50 mmHg.

GUIDELINES FOR ORGAN DONATION

Donor maintenance in the ICU

- Establish two reliable IV lines; one may be a central venous line.
- Try to maintain a systolic pressure above 90–100 mmHg to ensure adequate renal blood flow and urine output, by:
  - Giving a volume expander rapidly to restore blood pressure and maintain a CVP of 8–10 mmHg. Patients who have been dehydrated should receive 5% glucose or Hartmann's solution according to the plasma electrolyte results.
  - If hypotension is refractory and CVP >10, dobutamine 5–15 μg/kg/min should be started. Norepinephrine (see dose in page 12) may be added if systolic pressure remains <80 mmHg. A pulmonary artery flotation catheter may be useful.
- Insert a urinary catheter, maintain a urine output of at least 1.0 mL/kg/h:
  - Dopamine 2 μg/kg/min + mannitol 0.2 g/kg/h should be given, if oliguria persists.
  - If there is no response to the above measures, give furosemide (0.2 mg/kg IV) every 30 min (up to four doses).
  - Just before kidney donation, increase the urine output to 2–3 mL/kg/h using mannitol or furosemide.
- If diabetes insipidus (urine output > 4 mL/kg/h) develops, then give vasopressin (DDAVP) 2 μg subcutaneous or IV by infusion at 1 μg/h (0.02 μg/kg/h in children). Replacement during polyuria should be with 4% glucose/0.18% saline, if serum sodium is normal or with 5% glucose, if serum sodium is elevated. KCl 10–15 mmol/L may need to be added.
- Monitor arterial blood gases:
  - Adjust F_iO_2 to maintain a P_aO_2 >10 kPa.
  - Adjust ventilation to maintain a P_aCO_2 of 5 kPa.
- Monitor blood glucose concentration hourly. If the concentration increases above 6 mmol/L, start an insulin infusion.
- Aim to keep body temperature at 34–36°C and Hb >10 g/dL.
- The following may be asked for certain patients: ABO blood group, plasma urea and electrolytes, viral hepatitis serology and HIV status, ABGs, liver function tests, tissue type, ECG, CXR and serum amylase.

Absolute contraindications to organ donation

The only absolute contraindication is a transmissible infection for which there is no cure (e.g. CJD, HIV). All other patients should be referred to the transplant co-ordinator.

Some organs can be retrieved from non-heart beating donors. Criteria for this are as follows:

- <65 years old,
- no damage to organs.

Cases normally referred to the Coroner

All deaths from

- accidents or misadventure;
- abortions;
- alcoholism;
- anaesthetics (death resulting any time after the administration of the anaesthetic and before recovering from the effects of it);
- drugs, therapeutic or of addiction;
- industrial diseases;
- medical mishaps;
- pensioners (service disability);
- poisoning;
- prisoners – including any person in the custody of the police;
- any death of which the cause is unknown or in doubt;
- any death which cannot be certified as a natural one by a registered medical practitioner who attended the deceased for a reasonable period before death;
- death in the course of a surgical operation must always be reported to the Coroner. When the operation is for natural disease, it is normally accepted, subject to enquiry, that the cause of death was the disease and not the operation.

Pathology Handbook. Addenbrooke's Hospital NHS Trust. 1999.

CLASSIFICATION SYSTEMS

GLASGOW COMA SCALE

Sum of best eye-opening, best verbal and best motor responses. It cannot be applied to pre-verbal children, patients who are hypoxic, shocked, intoxicated, receiving neuromuscular-blocking agents or sedatives or those with a cervical cord lesion.

Eyes open	
Never	1
To pain	2
To speech	3
Spontaneously	4
Best verbal responses	
None	1
Garbled/incomprehensible sounds	2
Inappropriate words	3
Confused but converses	4
Oriented	5
Best motor responses	
None	1
Extension (decerebrate rigidity)	2
Abnormal flexion (decorticate rigidity)	3
Withdrawal	4
Localises pain	5
Obeys commands	6
Total	3–15

Teasdale G, Jennett B. Assessment of coma and impaired consciousness. *Lancet* 1974; **2**: 81–84

MODIFIED NEW YORK HEART ASSOCIATION (NYHA) FUNCTIONAL CLASSIFICATION OF HEART DISEASE

Class I	Asymptomatic except during severe exertion
Class II	Symptomatic with moderate activity
Class III	Symptomatic with minimal activity
Class IV	Symptomatic at rest

ASA CLASSIFICATION OF PHYSICAL STATUS

Class I	Normal healthy patient
Class II	A patient with mild systemic disease and no functional limitations
Class III	A patient with moderate to severe systemic disease that results in some functional limitation
Class IV	A patient with severe systemic disease that is a constant threat to life and functionally incapacitating
Class V	Moribund patient not expected to survive 24 h with or without surgery
Class VI	A brain-death patient, whose organs are being retrieved

American Society of Anesthesiologists: New classification of physical status. *Anesthesiology* 1963; **24**: 111

Emergency operation: the symbol 'E' is appended to the appropriate classification

ADDENBROOKE'S SEDATION SCORE

1	Agitated
2	Awake
3	Roused by voice
4	Roused by tracheal suction
5	Unrousable
6	Paralysed
7	Asleep
In pain	Y/N
Tolerant of ventilator	Y/N

RAMSAY SEDATION SCORE

Awake levels

1	Patient anxious and agitated or restless
2	Patient co-operative, oriented and tranquil
3	Patient responds to command only

Asleep levels (response to glabellar tap or auditory stimulus)

4	Brisk response
5	Sluggish response
6	No response

Ramsay MA, Savege TM, Simpson BR, et al. Controlled sedation with alphaxalone – alphadolone. *BMJ* 1974; **2**: 656–659

APACHE II: A SEVERITY OF DISEASE CLASSIFICATION SYSTEM

	High-abnormal range					Low-abnormal range			
	+4	+3	+2	+1	0	+1	+2	+3	+4
Physiological variable									
Temperature – rectal (°C)	≥41	39–40.9		38.5–38.9	36–38.4	34–35.9	32–33.9	30–31.9	≤29.9
Mean arterial pressure (mmHg)	≥160	130–159	110–129		70–109		50–69		≤49
Heart rate (ventricular response)	≥180	140–179	110–139		70–109		55–69	40–54	≤39
Respiratory rate (non-ventilated or ventilated)	≥50	35–49		25–34	12–24	10–11	6–9		≤5
Oxygenation: If F_IO_2 ≥ 0.5 record A–aDO2	≥500	350–499	200–349	<200					
If sFO_2 ≤ 0.5 record only P_aO_2 (mmHg)					>70	61–70		55–60	<55

	+4	+3	+2	+1	0	+1	+2	+3	+4
Arterial pH	≥7.7	7.6–7.69		7.5–7.59	7.33–7.49		7.25–7.32	7.15–7.24	<7.15
Serum sodium (mmol/L)	≥180	160–179	155–159	150–154	130–149		120–129	111–119	≤110
Serum potassium (mmol/L)	≥7	6–6.9		5.5–5.9	3.5–5.4	3.0–3.4	2.5–2.9		<2.5
Serum creatinine (μmol/L)	≥300	171–299	121–170		50–120		<50		
Haematocrit (%)	≥60		50–59.9	46–49.9	30–45.9		20–29.9		<20
White blood count (×1000/mm³)	≥40		20–39.9	15–19.9	3–14.9		1–2.9		<1

Glasgow coma score (GCS): score = 15 − actual GCS

Age points

Age (years)	≤44	45–54	55–64	65–74	≥75
Points	0	2	3	5	6

Chronic health points

Two points for elective post-operative admission, or five points if emergency operation or non-operative admission, if patient has significant chronic liver, cardiovascular, respiratory or renal disease, or is immunocompromised.

Knaus WA, Draper EA, Wagner DP, Zimmerman JE. APACHE II: a severity of disease classification system. *Crit Care Med* 1985; **13**: 818–829

NATIONAL BODIES IN ANAESTHESIA AND SPECIALIST SOCIETIES

Anaesthetic Research Society
Tel: 0115 970 9229
Fax: 0115 970 0739
www.ars.ac.uk

Association of Anaesthetists of Great Britain and Ireland
Tel: 020 7631 1650
www.aagbi.org

Association of Cardiothoracic Anaesthetists
Tel: 020 8980 4433
Fax: 020 8983 2411
www.acta.org.uk

Association of Paediatric Anaesthetists (Great Britain and Ireland)
Tel: 01603 287 086
Fax: 01603 287 886
www.apagbi.org.uk

British Association of Immediate Care (Basics)
Tel: 0870 1654 999
Fax: 0870 1654 949
www.basics.org.uk

Faculty of Anaesthetists of the Royal College of Surgeons of Ireland
Tel: 00 353166 14412

Intensive Care Society
Tel: 020 7631 8890
Fax: 020 7631 8897
www.ics.ac.uk

Obstetric Anaesthetists Association
Tel: 020 8741 1311
Fax: 020 8741 0611
www.oaa-anaes.ac.uk

Paediatric Intensive Care Society
Tel: 0114 2717 494
www.ukpicu.com

Pain Society
Tel: 020 7631 8870
www.painsociety.org

Association of Burns and Reconstructive Anaesthetists
Tel: 01245 516 241
Fax: 01245 516 244
www.abra.org.uk

Resuscitation Council (UK)
Tel: 020 7388 4678
Fax: 020 7383 0773
www.resus.org.uk

Royal College of Anaesthetists
Tel: 020 7908 7300
www.rcoa.ac.uk

Royal Society of Medicine (Section of Anaesthetics)
Tel: 020 7290 2986
Fax: 020 7290 2989
www.rsm.ac.uk

World Federation of Societies of Anaesthesiologists
Tel: 020 7836 5652

BIBLIOGRAPHY

A Guide to Antibiotic Therapy in Adult Patients. Addenbrooke's Hospital NHS Trust. December 2001

Aitkenhead AR, Rowbotham DJ and Smith G. *Textbook of Anaesthesia*, fourth edition. Churchill Livingstone, London. 2001

Bingham R, Handley A, Evans T, Nolan J, Phillips B, Richmond S and Wyllie J. *Resuscitation Guidelines*. Resuscitation Council, London. 2000

Brower RG, Matthay MA, Morris A, Schoenfeld D, Thompson BT and Wheeler A. Ventilation with lower tidal volumes as compared with traditional tidal volumes for acute lung injury and the acute respiratory distress syndrome. *New Engl J Med* 2000; **342**: 1301–8

Cerra FB, Rios M, Blackburn GL, Irwin RS, Jeejeebhoy K, Katz DP, Pingleton SK, Pomposelli J, Rombeau JL, Shronts E, Wolfe RR and Zaloga GP. Applied nutrition in ICU patients – a consensus statement of the American College of Chest Physicians. *Chest* 1997; **111**: 769–78

Checklist for Anaesthetic Apparatus. Association of Anaesthetists of Great Britain and Ireland, London. 1997. www.aagbi.org/guidelines.html

Irwin RS, Cerra FB and Rippe JM. *Intensive Care Medicine*, fourth edition. Lippincott-Raven Publishers, Philadelphia. 1999

Malignant Hyperthermia. Association of Anaesthetists in Great Britain and Ireland. 1998. www.aagbi.org/guidelines.html

Miller RD. *Anesthesia,* fifth edition. Churchill Livingstone, Philadelphia, Pennsylvania. 2000

Morgan GE, Mikhail MS and Murray MJ. *Clinical Anesthesiology,* third edition. International Edition. McGraw-Hill, USA. 2002

Park GR and Sladen RN. *Top Tips in Critical Care,* first edition. Greenwich Medical Media Limited, London. 2001

Pathology Handbook. Addenbrooke's Hospital NHS Trust. 1999

Recommendations for Standards of Monitoring during Anaesthesia and Recovery. Association of Anaesthetists of Great Britain and Ireland, London. 2000. www.aagbi.org/guidelines.html

Special Issue Guidelines 2000 for cardiopulmonary resuscitation and emergency cardiovascular care – an international consensus on science. *Resuscitation* 2000; **46**(1–3): 135–53, 185–93

Sumner E and Hatch DJ. *Paediatric Anaesthesia,* second edition. Arnold publishers, London. 2000

Suspected Anaphylactic Reactions Associated with Anaesthesia, revised edition. Association of Anaesthetists in Great Britain and Ireland. 1995. www.aagbi.org/guidelines.html

Van Den Berghe G, Wouters P and Weekers F. Intensive insulin therapy in critically ill patients. *New Engl J Med* 2001; **345**: 1359–67

Webb AR, Shapiro MJ, Singer M and Suter PM. *Oxford Textbook of Critical Care,* first edition. Oxford University Press, Oxford. 1999